HOW TO LIVE ON DIET:
A guide on how to live a diet life without spending much.

James walter

Table of content

Chapter 1

WHAT IS YOUR PHILOSOPHY?

"The philosophy of life leads to the fear of death. A man who lives completely is always ready to pass away!

I asked myself: What if you were asked, "What is your life philosophy?" during an interview? How quickly could you respond to such inquiry?

A conceptual framework for comprehending how the world functions and how you fit into the world is what I mean when I say "philosophy of life." The philosophy of life would address issues such as how you determine what is "good" and "bad," what success means, what your "mission" in life is (even if you don't believe there is one), if there is a God, how we should treat one another, etc.

You may refer to your way of life by any number of titles, including libertarian, feminist, liberal, conservative, Buddhist, Christian, entrepreneur, artist, environmentalist, tea party, and a host of others. Perhaps you believe that you could sum up your philosophy of life in one of those phrases, but for the most of us, I would venture to guess that our real philosophics arc more intricate and nuanced. They cannot be contained as readily. Could you explain yours to me if we had a conversation in person?

I believe I could categorize you readers into three categories based on what I know about you as a group.

The first group has a distinct life philosophy that you have carefully considered, put to the test, and routinely and openly utilize to direct your behavior. You are now known as "The True North Group." You have a compass for life, and you are aware of the real north, which is the direction that is correct. You could give me a clear, simple explanation of your philosophy of life if I requested you to do so right now. Even though you may not be able to describe it in a single word, you have given it some consideration and can explain why your philosophy of life makes sense to you and how it influences your mind. This is probably the smallest of the three groups.

The second category are those of you who have a loosely structured philosophy of life in which things fundamentally fit together, but which you couldn't explain quickly off the top of your head. If I gave you a little more time, you could come up with an overarching framework that covers most things, though the fringes and the corner cases of life would remain gray. I will call you "The Dusty Compass Group." It's like you have a compass for directing your life, but you forget to use it. You have a roughly coherent system for understanding the world, and you pretty much know it intuitively, but most of the time you don't explicitly use it to filter and direct your experience. The compass lies on the shelf collecting dust. When you eventually pull it out, you see it's gotten a little wacky and you need to recalibrate it. My guess is that this experience describes the largest group of people.

The third group I will call "The Inbox Group." For The Inbox Group I'm abandoning the compass metaphor because if you are in this group, you do not actually have a governing magnetic orientation for what life is about and where you are going. Life may be about something, heck, your life may be about something, but you don't know. You are too preoccupied to consider it. Your strategy, which mirrors how you handle email, is to just deal with what is presented to you. You get communications from people and organizations all the time trying to get your attention, and you essentially do what they say. Why do you watch that brand-new Netflix program? What makes you want to hear that brand-new Kanye song? In any case, why did you choose to become a surgeon? Actually, you don't know. The reasons you believe you know, though, turn out to be really flimsy. Though it could be the biggest, I believe this to be the second-largest group.

Members of these three groupings vary from one another virtually exclusively internally. They wouldn't be identifiable on the street. But they will have a very different subjective sense of life. One guy engages in squash because he adheres to the true north principle of pushing oneself to the maximum, taking care of one's health, and putting friendships with other players first. Another person could share your values but be unable to express them. He just knows that he enjoys playing. A third is just participating because someone asked him to. Perhaps all he wants is to be noticed at the racquet club. He could just like being questioned. While chasing a ball around a court is also an exterior activity, the mental drive and feeling are quite different.

I believe that living as a True North group member is preferable in general. In general, because there are some exclusions. Some individuals have very detailed life philosophies, but confining themselves to those concepts has left them unimaginative, uncurious, and a bit too self-assured that they know it all.

But generally speaking, I believe that having a clear plan for life and adhering to it are beneficial. If you stay modest, observant, and willing to be proven incorrect, True North is the way to proceed. The alternative to having an orienting vision for your life is becoming a member of the Dusty Compass Group or the Inbox Group. It implies that you continuously run the danger of losing sight of who you are, misinterpreting what life is all about, and veering off track (i.e., wasting your time).

The great leveler for these groupings is death. Even if you may spend the most of your time in the Dusty Compass Group or the Inbox Group, your life philosophy tends to become more pronounced when you get dangerously close to passing away—either your own death or the death of a loved one. Your experience of being on the verge of death serves as a shock that makes you wish to belong to the True North Group and to live, in a sense, on purpose. to make a difference.

It's possible that someone helped you with the practice of imagining what your obituary would say once you pass away. If we are being really honest, the way most of us are spending our time doesn't quite align with what we want our life to be about. It's like waking up from a fantasy to realize that.

The experience of being close to death for many of us causes us to turn away from "the things life is too short for" and toward the True North Group. When faced with death, we reflect carefully on what is important, and it should come as no surprise that family, friendships, treating others well, education, and maintaining our health top the list. We commit to making those things our top priorities. And we start to live more in accordance with our goals.

However, as the weeks and months pass, we begin to slip back to distraction gently, almost imperceptibly to us. We don't glance at the compass as much. We just respond to what is presented to us. Even if we are aware of what is essential to us, we often put it off until later. Although we don't fully forget what we believe life is all about, the idea gradually loses its clarity and poignancy, much like an old snapshot that has been exposed to the light. Without a defined philosophy of life to guide us, it is simple to follow the simplest path rather than leading lives that will leave a lasting impression on future generations.

I like to think of myself as a True North Guy, but in all honesty, I probably am more of a Dusty Compass with occasional forays into the True North. That is why I find it amazing when people manage to conduct their lives in accordance with their ideas. Because it is challenging to live with character, they are extraordinary. Living as though life is finite is difficult. And because of this, I sometimes find that contemplating death's truth is one of the finest things I can do to fully appreciate the reality of my existence.

Chapter 2

The History of longevity.

How long did humans live in the past? You often hear statistics about the average life span of people who lived hundreds, even thousands, of years ago. Were our ancestors really dying at the age of 30 or 40 back then? Here's a little primer on longevity throughout history to help you understand how life expectancy and life spans have changed over time.

This article will explain the average life span of people throughout history.

Two African women looking at photo album - stock photo

Life Span vs. Life Expectancy

The term life expectancy means the average lifespan of an entire population, taking into account all mortality figures for that specific group of people. Life span is a measure of the actual length of an individual's life.

While both terms seem straightforward, a lack of historical artifacts and records have made it challenging for researchers to determine how life spans have evolved throughout history.

The Definition of Life Span

The Life Span of Early Man

Until fairly recently, little information existed about how long prehistoric people lived. Having access to too few fossilized human remains made it difficult for historians to estimate the demographics of any population.

Anthropology professors Rachel Caspari and Sang-Hee Lee, of Central Michigan University and the University of California at Riverside, respectively, chose instead to analyze the relative ages of skeletons found in archeological digs in eastern and southern Africa, Europe, and elsewhere.[1]

After comparing the proportion of those who died young with those who died at an older age, the team concluded that longevity only began to significantly increase—that is, past the age of 30 or so—about 30,000 years ago, which is quite late in the span of human evolution.

In an article published in 2011 in Scientific American, Caspari calls the shift the "evolution of grandparents." It marks the first time in human history that three generations might have co-existed.[2]

Ancient Through Pre-Industrial Times

Life expectancy estimates that describe the population as a whole also suffer from a lack of reliable evidence gathered from these periods.

In a 2010 article published in the Proceedings of the National Academy of Sciences, gerontologist and evolutionary biologist Caleb Finch describes the average life spans in ancient Greek and Roman times as short at approximately of 20 to 35 years, though he laments these numbers are based on "notoriously unrepresentative" graveyard epitaphs and samples.3

Moving forward along the historic timeline, Finch lists the challenges of deducing historic life spans and causes of death in this information vacuum.

As a kind of research compromise, he and other evolution experts suggest a reasonable comparison can be made with demographic data from pre-industrial Sweden (mid-18th century) and certain contemporary, small, hunter-gatherer societies in countries like Venezuela and Brazil.3

Finch writes that judging by this data the main causes of death during these early centuries would most certainly have been infections, whether from infectious diseases or infected wounds resulting from accidents or fighting.

Unhygienic living conditions and little access to effective medical care meant life expectancy was likely limitcd to about 35 years of age. That's life expectancy at birth, a figure dramatically influenced by infant mortality—pegged at the time as high as 30%.

It does not mean that the average person living in 1200 A.D. died at the age of 35. Rather, for every child that died in infancy, another person might have lived to see their 70th birthday.

Early years up to the age of about 15 continued to be perilous, thanks to risks posed by disease, injuries, and accidents. People who survived this hazardous period of life could well make it into old age.

Other infectious diseases like cholera, tuberculosis, and smallpox would go on to limit longevity, but none on a scale quite as damaging of the bubonic plague in the 14th century. The Black Plague moved through Asia and Europe, and wiped out as much as a third of Europe's population, temporarily shifting life expectancy downward.

 An Overview of Bubonic Plague
From the 1800s to Today
From the 1500s onward, till around the year 1800, life expectancy throughout Europe hovered between 30 and 40 years of age.

Since the early 1800s, Finch writes that life expectancy at birth has doubled in a period of only 10 or so generations. Improved health care, sanitation, immunizations, access to clean running water, and better nutrition are all credited with the massive increase.

Though it's hard to imagine, doctors only began regularly washing their hands before surgery in the mid-1800s. A better understanding of hygiene and the transmission of microbes has since contributed substantially to public health.

Disease was still common, however, and impacted life expectancy. Parasites, typhoid, and infections like rheumatic fever and scarlet fever were all common during the 1800s.

The History of Surgery: A Timeline of Medicine

Even as recently as 1921, countries like Canada still had an infant mortality rate of about 10%, meaning 1 out of every 10 babies did not survive. According to Statistics Canada, this meant a life expectancy or average survival rate in that country that was higher at age 1 than at birth—a condition that persisted right until the early 1980s.

Today most industrialized countries boast life expectancy figures of more than 75 years, according to comparisons compiled by the Central Intelligence Agency.
In the Future
Some researchers have predicted that lifestyle factors like obesity will halt or even reverse the rise in life expectancy for the first time in modern history.
Epidemiologists and gerontologists such as S. Jay Olshanky warn that in the United States—where two-thirds of the population is overweight or obese—obesity and its complications, like diabetes, could very well reduce life expectancy at all ages in the first half of 21st century.

In the meantime, rising life expectancy in the West brings both good and bad news—it's nice to be living longer, but you are now more vulnerable to the types of illnesses that hit as you get older. These age-related diseases include coronary artery disease, certain cancers, diabetes, and dementia.

While they can affect quantity and quality of life, many of these conditions can be prevented or at least delayed through healthy lifestyle choices like following an anti-aging diet, maintaining a healthy weight, exercising regularly and keeping stress hormones.

Chapter 3

Weight loss with the longevity diet

The benefits of weight loss to health and longevity are well-documented. The steps taken towards weight loss can be beneficial within themselves; for example, exercise promotes holistic health, especially cardiovascular health, while eating an optimal diet of grains, legumes, fish, fruit, and vegetables can improve longevity by 10 years!

This can be supported by taking longevity supplements, which contain active ingredients that work on the body's aging pathways. Some versions even have additional weight loss benefits, like GLYLO's glycation longevity supplements, which apply research from the Buck Institute. However, these supplements should only be taken to complement a healthy lifestyle for longevity.

Weight loss itself can have further benefits to longevity; one study found that intentional weight loss reduced the risk of all-cause mortality in unhealthy and obese adults.

The greatest benefit was seen in those with obesity-related mctabolic illnesses like diabetes and hypertension, as well as at-risk ethnic groups.

Whether the long-term effect of weight loss benefits longevity in those of a healthy weight remains less conclusive. One study into the effects of weight loss on all-cause mortality found that while intentional weight loss benefited longevity in obese and at-risk people, the effects in healthy people of normal weight were negligible. Indeed, unintentional weight loss in this group may be a symptom of the disease and can predict mortality risk as we age.

One explanation for this difference between groups may be that obese people are more motivated to make a change like reducing fat intake or increasing exercise level, benefiting their holistic health. In people of a healthy weight, weight loss through energy restriction may result in loss of lean body mass rather than body fat. It is hypothesized that fat loss can reduce all-cause mortality while loss of lean body mass could increase it

While moderate weight loss in people of healthy weight appears to have a negligible, and possibly even negative, impact on longevity, losing weight in obese and at-risk people can benefit health and longevity. This supports the general hypothesis that the most effective way to guarantee your future longevity is through the tried and tested method of a healthy, balanced diet alongside regular exercise.

Chapter 4

Reasons for diet failure .

According to the experts, these are the four leading causes of diet dropout:

1. **Choosing the Wrong Diet**

Choosing a restrictive diet that doesn't fit your lifestyle is a major reason for giving up on weight loss efforts, says Holly Wyatt, MD, Colorado University's program director for obesity research and education. When the diet is too difficult in the first place, sustaining it long-term will be almost impossible. Boredom factor and all it takes is one misstep to cause a dieter to give up.

"There is no one perfect diet that is the best," says Wyatt. "Instead, look for a sound diet plan that you can live with, day in and day out." It should also allow you to enjoy small portions of your favorite foods.

Diet Success Tip: Diets that work are diets that last. Don't think of your eating plan as a "diet" you can go on and off of. Choose a health plan that fits your lifestyle -- one that you can see following for the rest of your life.

Successful losers understand that whether they're trying to lose weight or maintain the lost weight, theirs is a lifestyle of constant vigilance.

"Losing weight and maintaining it is among the most difficult things people can do because it has no end," says Gary Foster, Ph.D., director of the Center for Obesity Research and Education at Temple

University in Philadelphia. "To succeed is to make the vigilance part of a regular lifestyle."

2. Unrealistic Expectations

Failing to lose weight quickly enough is the Achilles heel of most dieters, says Champagne. Weight loss may take longer than anticipated, or your diet may need adjustments along the way.

"Most dieters want to lose large amounts of weight and aren't happy unless they lose 30%-40%" of their body weight, says Wyatt.

When you set the bar unrealistically high, she says, it can feel like you failed when you don't meet your goals. And when you think of yourself as a failure, this can trigger a return to old eating habits.

Diet Success Tip: You might not fit into those skinny jeans, but keep in mind that losing even a little weight goes a long way toward improving your health. Research has shown that losing 10% of your body weight (for example, going from 200 to 180 pounds) can have big payoffs for your health.

"Medically, 10% weight loss can lower blood pressure, cholesterol [and] triglyceride levels, improve glucose sensitivity and sleep apnea," says Wyatt.

In addition, it can help you feel better about yourself.

3. Dieting Without Exercise

Some people just don't like to exercise or have physical limitations that prevent them from doing it. But if you don't want to be a diet drop-out, you need to find some form of physical activity you can do most days of the week.

"If there is one behavior that predicts weight loss success, it is being physically active regularly," says Foster.

Further, physical activity brings many health and psychological benefits aside from weight loss.

Diet Success Tip: Exercise does not have to happen in a gym - try gardening, dancing, walking, bike riding, or playing tennis, whatever you enjoy. Start slowly and gradually increase your intensity. Check with your doctor if you have physical limitations. Working out in the pool, for example, cushions joints and adds the extra benefit of water resistance. One of the simplest and easiest ways to exercise is to trap on a pedometer and count your steps throughout the day, aiming for 10,000 each day.

4. **Not Changing Your Environment**

Willpower alone won't cut it. To be a successful loser, you need to create a diet-friendly environment at home, at work, and socially.

"It is hard to continually push away from the wings at happy hour, candy on your desk, or a house full of temptations. If you want to succeed, you need to make changes in your environment so you are not constantly dealing with or resisting temptations," says Wyatt.

When you can't eat the same things as your friends, or your family doesn't support your weight-loss efforts, this makes dieting more difficult, says Champagne.

Diet Success Tip: Seek support from your family, friends, and co-workers. And, Wyatt suggests, remove temptations wherever you can. Stock your kitchen with nutritious foods so you have ingredients on hand for healthy meals and snacks. Take nutritious snacks and meals with you when you're on the go so you'll be prepared when hunger strikes. Remove the candy dish from your desk, skip happy hour with your friends -- do whatever it takes to set yourself up for success, even if it means hanging around with differe.

Chapter 5

How to succeed

For the majority of people, making healthy, long-term lifestyle changes is the best way to lose weight. Fad diets and "how to lose weight quickly" plans may help you lose weight quickly, but they are frequently unhealthy and ultimately ineffective.

Consider how frequently you have enrolled in the newest weight loss fad only to experience fleeting results and end up gaining all the weight back after a few weeks. No fun. not good for you

Here are some suggestions for losing weight that might enable you to reach a healthy weight:

1. ***Moving forward***: Regular exercise is one of the best ways to lose weight.
The great thing about exercise is that you can find a form you like because there are so many different kinds of it. Running, walking the dog, playing tennis, swimming, hiking, or lifting weights in the gym all burn calories and build muscle.
Additionally, adding muscle will increase your resting metabolism, or how quickly your body burns calories while at rest. Additionally, you'll increase your serotonin levels, which will make you happier and less likely to overeat.

Here are some of the best workouts to lose weight:

Hit Training: high-intensity interval training is one of the best things you can do to burn fat and lose weight. It requires you to work at a high level of intensity and use a wide range of muscles for a short time and is followed by a brief rest period. Try this 15-minute HIIT workout plan you can do at home.

Weightlifting: building muscle often produces fat loss and some people prefer weight training to cardio – who doesn't want to feel strong?! You can start with light weights and increase them when you're used to them and they become easy to lift. Here are some of the best exercises to lose weight.

Remember: if you are weight training or starting a new exercise regime, your body will likely cling to some water weight, at least in the beginning, which can make the scale go up. Building muscle doesn't always result in weight loss either – but you may lose inches.

This is because 1lb of muscle will take up less room than 1lb of fat, yet they weigh the same. Try taking measurements of your waist, hips, chest, and other areas so you have non-scale ways to track your progress.

2. **Base your weight loss diet around healthy choices**

The best diet for weight loss should act as a stepping stone to a healthier lifestyle. But it can seem like quite a daunting and difficult task to figure out what to eat to lose weight. It shouldn't be hard though and you don't have to follow an elaborate or expensive diet to lose weight.

You may begin to make healthy decisions by increasing your intake of complex carbs, lean proteins, fruits, and vegetables, as well as other foods that are proven to help you lose weight. You can also cut down on alcohol and other "treats," and increase your exercise.

If you do this and don't lose any weight, fat, or inches, you may need to actively cut back on calories or increase your activity. Both of these actions ensure that your body burns more calories each day than you consume.

4. **Quit estimating serving sizes**.

You will always gain weight if you eat too much. So that you always have food on hand that is prepared to consume in the proper portions when you are hungry, stock your kitchen ahead of time with portioned items in serving containers.

To assist you to comprehend the quantities you should be consuming and the nutrients they contain, you may also spend money on some food scales.

5. **Mindful eating**

It's a good idea to pay attention to your food while you're eating mindfully. Take a little pause and concentrate on your sensation of satisfaction while you eat. When you are full, this aids in turning down the hunger center in the brain, making weight loss easier.

6. **Pay attention to your body.**

Don't skip breakfast if you're hungry in the morning simply because you've heard it would make you lose weight. In the same vein, resist the urge to push down a large breakfast, or any meal, for that matter.

Eat when you're hungry and stop when you're full to eat instinctively. Do it if it means eating supper at 8 o'clock. You will lose weight, fat, or inches as long as you are burning more calories than you are taking in.

7. **Establish a routine**

You could feel fuller for longer by eating at regular intervals throughout the day, which might help you avoid mindless snacking.

8. **Consume fruit and vegetables**.

Fruit and veg are some of the best foods to eat to lose weight. The majority of our favorite fruits are rich in vitamins and minerals and low in calories and fat. To bulk out your meals and see whether they may take the place of your unhealthy snacks, be sure to include them in your daily diet. Dried fruit is easy and a fantastic snack.

9. **Choose meals rich in fiber**.

You may feel fuller for longer by eating fiber-rich foods including fruit and vegetables, wholegrain bread, oats, brown rice and pasta, peas and lentils, and beans. By including these items throughout your meals, you should be able to avoid snacking and nighttime cravings.

Did you realize? The water-soluble fiber glucomannan, which swells in the stomach to make people feel full, is used to help individuals lose weight. You may consume it as a drink or as rice or other favorite carbohydrates in diet form.

Decide on a smaller plate.

You could find portion management to be simpler if you use smaller dishes and bowls for your meals. A full bowl of food is often far more fulfilling for most individuals than a smaller-than-usual piece on a big plate.

Did you realize? Eating more slowly may be essential for weight reduction since it takes your stomach 20 minutes to signal your brain that it is full.

11. Avoid imposing food bans

Foods that you enjoy but that are 'unhealthy' will likely make you crave them more if you forbid them. If a treat fits within your daily calorie budget, there is no reason why you can't have it occasionally. It's preferable to occasionally splurge on the foods you enjoy rather than forbidding them and then bingeing on them.

So feel free to indulge in that dessert or takeout whenever you want. It all comes down to striking a balance between the foods you eat and the exercise you get in.

12. **Avoid buying junk food in bulk.**
Get some healthy snacks in the house instead of keeping a pantry stocked with tempting junk food like chocolate, chips, and biscuits. Instead, keep some popcorn, fruit juice, fruit, oat cakes, rice cakes, and other wholesome snacks on hand for those times when you get the munchies.

13. **Reduce your alcohol consumption**

Do you know the caloric content of your favorite alcoholic beverages? They occasionally contain more than just a typical chocolate bar! So, when you're trying to lose weight, it's a good idea to keep this in mind. Alcohol is unlikely to help and just adds to your daily calories in a big way. However, if you do fancy a drink, stick to clear spirits for a lower-calorie option. G & 'slimline T' anybody?

14. **Drink lots of water**

Find yourself feeling hungry when you've not long catcn a mcal. Sometimes we feel hungry when we are dehydrated. 9 The best thing to do is try to stay hydrated all day so we don't confuse the two and overeat when a glass of water is what we wanted.

15. Get lean with coffee

Research has revealed those taking a green coffee bean extract lost just over a stone, or 10 percent of their body weight. It's thought a compound called chlorogenic acid, found in the unroasted beans, may influence glucose and fat metabolism.

The caffeine in cups of coffee may help you to lose weight too. Try swapping your lattes and cappuccinos for americanos or filter coffees to cut down on calories while still enjoying the energy boost and potential weight loss benefits.

Get sipping and see what weight loss coffee benefits you discover!

16. **Check out the green tea weight loss benefits**:

Numerous studies have shown green tea can help you lose weight. It's thought the fragrant cuppa could help the body burn calories and fat. What's not to like?!

17. **Try a fat burner**

A fat burner could be a useful addition to your weight loss regimen if you are doing all of the aforementioned things and want to lose weight quickly. Utilizing natural substances and stimulants that could increase calorie burn together with a good diet and exercise plan, fat burners are items that might assist in speed weight reduction.

www.ingramcontent.com/pod-product-compliance
Lightning Source LLC
Chambersburg PA
CBHW070226260726
48658CB00006BA/2191